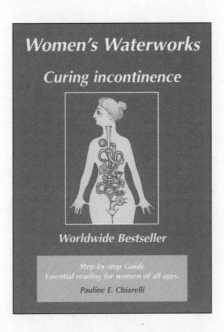

Women's Waterworks

Curing incontinence

Worldwide Bestseller

Step-by-step Guide
Essential reading for women of all ages.
Pauline E. Chiarelli

**There's a one-in-three chance that any woman has a secret – incontinence – the problem of being unable to control her waterworks. The real shame is not that she actually has this problem, but that it can be prevented.
Step by step, in everyday language, this book shows the effective way of curing the problem, no matter how old a woman may be.**

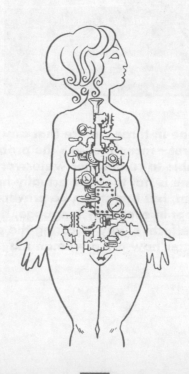

ABOUT THE AUTHOR

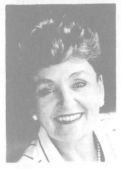

Pauline Chiarelli is a consultant physiotherapist and continence adviser who has wide experience as a general physiotherapist. Her early professional experience in the field of prenatal education led to an interest in training/retraining the muscles of the pelvic floor. A widespread lack of information about treatment for these muscles led to more and more calls for Pauline to share her experiences and treatment protocols with other physiotherapists. It soon became evident that specialised knowledge about urinary continence would be necessary if she were to be able to answer all the questions that started coming her way. Studies in the United Kingdom and Australia have provided the basis for her efforts in continence promotion. Pauline has led many seminars not only for professionals but also for ordinary people whose overwhelming need for information led her to write this book. She travels widely and has appeared in a number of international forums on continence as well as being a sought-after media speaker. Pauline has a Masters degree in medical science in the field of health promotion and is currently working toward her Ph.D. She lives in Australia with her husband and family.

DEDICATION

I dedicate this book to my husband George, who is teaching me to accept the things I cannot change, encouraging me to change the things I can, and helping me towards the wisdom to know the difference.

ACKNOWLEDGEMENTS

I would like to acknowledge the support given to me over many years by Dr Richard Millard – Consultant Urologist, Prince Henry Hospital, Sydney – without whose help women's waterworks would still be a mystery to me. Also, the Australian Physiotherapy Association, NSW Branch, especially the Continence and Women's Health Special Group within it, for helping me to promote the physiotherapy profession as a moving force (pardon the pun) in the treatment of the muscles of the pelvic floor.

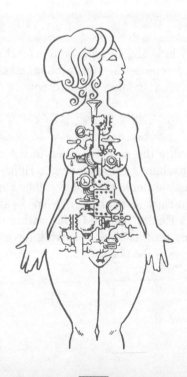

CONTENTS

Published by Gore & Osment Publications
Postal address:
80-82 McLachlan Avenue
Rushcutters Bay NSW 2011
Australia
Telephone: (02) 9361 6366
Fax: (02) 9360 7558

© **Pauline E. Chiarelli 1992**
National Library of Australia Cataloguing-in-Publication entry
**Chiarelli, Pauline E
Women's Waterworks
Curing Incontinence**
ISBN 1 875531 00 9.
1. Urinary incontinence
2. Urinary incontinence – Treatment I. Title.
616.63

Author
Pauline Chiarelli M.A.P.A.
Production Editor/Design
Sheridan Packer
Concept Design
Stephen Joseph
Sub Editor
Linda Drummond
Illustrations
Brendan Akhurst
Marketing Director
Stephen Balme

First published 1988
Reprinted 1989, 1990, 1991, 1992, 1993, 1995, 1996, 1998, 2001

© Gore & Osment Publications Pty Ltd (ACN 052 893 188) an imprint of J.B. Fairfax Press Pty Limited (ACN 003 738 430), 80-82 McLachlan Avenue, Rushcutters Bay NSW 2011.

Printed by Griffin Press Pty Ltd Netley, SA

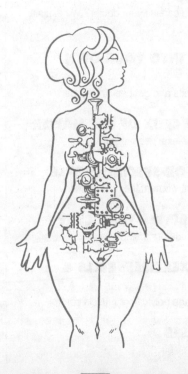

CHAPTER 1

INTRODUCING WOMEN'S WATERWORKS

T here's a one in three chance that any woman has a secret: incontinence, the problem of being unable to always control her waterworks. Chances are, too, that if she has been brave enough to confide this secret (maybe to her mother or best friend), she was sympathetically consoled and told: "That's okay, I leak too. It's part of the price women pay for being mothers". This reasoning is used so often that it has been accepted as fact, but take heart, there's no truth behind it at all. Leakage may be common, but it's never normal. And, more importantly, incontinence is curable. Leakage is so common that it's not unusual for every member of a women's senior basketball team or social tennis group to wear protective pads during games. Some women limit their golf games to nine holes or visit the 'ladies' whenever the clubhouse comes into view. Others take up swimming for exercise and avoid aerobic classes, jogging or power walking just to keep the secret of their leakage safe.

The onset of this embarrassing problem is very gradual, but never unnoticed. It's your body's way of telling you that things are not quite as they should be. Take it from me, leaking urine is neither normal or acceptable and your little secret is really just the beginning of what can become a downward spiral where loss of bladder control goes hand-in-hand with loss of self respect as well as anxiety and depression ... extra burdens you can certainly do without. Around thirty five per cent of women over the age of 65 years suffer incontinence and the real shame is not that they actually have this problem, but that it can be prevented. The easiest time to regain control of your waterworks is when you first start to notice leakage. This initial leaking, called "stress incontinence", is caused by a weakening of the muscles that keep urine stored in the bladder. These muscles, known as the pelvic floor muscles, fail to

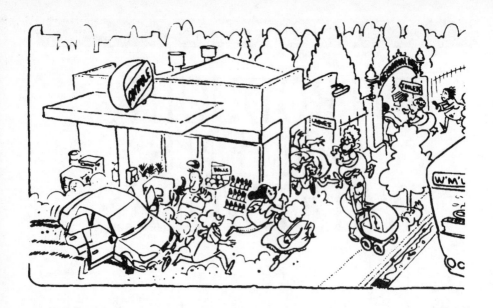

fight the forces which push down from the abdomen when you laugh, sneeze, run, jump or perform any other type of physical exertion.

Sound familiar? If unchecked, simple stress incontinence can progress to include symptoms such as urgency and frequency in the following way: you're running to reach the bank before closing time and suddenly you feel dampness spreading between your legs. You divert to the nearest toilet to check that there are no tell-take wet patches on your clothes. You don't really feel the need to, but you go to the toilet just to make sure the leak doesn't happen again. Anxiety sets in and, whenever you think there is the slightest possibility of a re-run, you take yourself off to the toilet to empty your bladder, establishing a pattern of frequency. Soon you are a confirmed toilet hopper: you know every 'ladies' in town and which service stations along your usual driving routes have public conveniences. You cut down on fluid intake. You start joking about your weak bladder and friends all laugh in a supporting, sympathetic way. They either share your problem or know someone who does, so acceptance of the situation leads to the belief that it's okay.

This is just not so! The purpose of this book is to help you regain control of your waterworks so there are no leakages and no frequent dashes to the toilet. Your bladder will no longer be a bossy dictator telling you that you need to urinate every half hour. To take charge again, you need to understand how the waterworks function and why the system breaks down. When women's waterworks break down they usually complain of three main symptoms:

• Stress Incontinence; the leaks which happen when they cough, sneeze, swing at a golf ball or lunge at tennis.

• Urgency; the really strong need to pass urine which, if ignored, most women

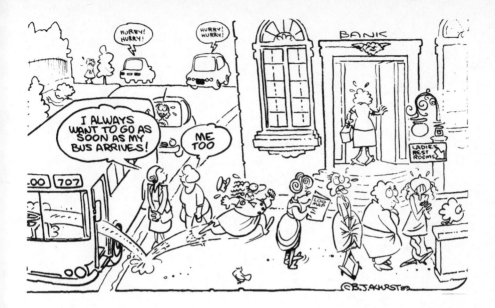

feel would cause them to wet their pants.

• Frequency; the need to empty the bladder often, with only a short time between visits to the toilet. If this frequency occurs during the night it is referred to as nocturia.

A combination of any or all of these symptoms can be present.

Do You Have A Problem?

Most women consider their toilet habits 'normal'. But are they?

• Do you go to the toilet six to eight times each day only?
• Do you sleep through or get up only once through the night?
• Do you have dry pants at all times?
• Do you pass 300 - 400mls each time? (one coffee mug holds 250mls)
• Do you pass water easily, without straining or stopping and starting?
• Do you find urinating is painless and quite a comfortable thing to do?

If you answered yes to all these questions, you have no problem, your urinary pattern is normal.

If you have answered no to any of these questions then something in your waterworks is not quite right and you should take steps right now to help overcome these problems before they become worse. Otherwise, the chance of being an elderly incontinent women is a real one. Although family carers may put up with a lot while looking after elderly relatives, incontinence is often the straw that breaks the camel's back, so to speak. It is thought that up to sixty per cent of all people in nursing homes are there not because they have decreased mental faculties or because they have lost the ability to move around, but because they are incontinent.

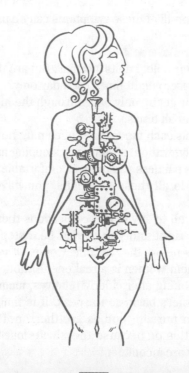

CHAPTER 2

WHAT WE'VE GOT AND HOW IT WORKS

The waterworks are easiest to understand if you think of the bladder as a reservoir which is filled slowly but constantly by the kidneys from above, in much the same way as a dam is filled by a river. When the storage in the bladder reaches a certain level, the 'hold on' mechanisms let go and urine is pushed out until the bladder is empty. The 'hold on' mechanisms take over again and the bladder slowly fills once more. Simple, isn't it?

The Bladder

This is a hollow muscular pump which sits just behind the pubic bone - the hard bone you can feel beneath your pubic hair. Unless your bladder is full, you should not be able to feel it. The kidneys feed urine into the bladder via tubes called ureters. The bladder empties out via another tube known as the urethra and through the perineum (the area between your legs). The bladder muscle itself is called the detrusor muscle. It's very important to understand that urine does not run out – it's actually pushed out by the detrusor muscle of the bladder as it contracts. You have no voluntary control over the contraction of your detrusor muscle.

Stopping the leaks is actually the job of your pelvic floor muscles and your urethral sphincter. Both of these are under your voluntary control. The urethral sphincter is like the string in a drawstring purse. It holds on all day and your pelvic floor muscles help it to hold on tight when you cough, sneeze, laugh or run. This usually happens without you thinking about it. It happens as a reflex, just a split second before you cough or laugh. The urethral sphincter mechanism squeezes the urethra shut and stops the urine escaping from the bladder. Each time it does this, however, it achieves another much less

The Muscles of the Pelvic Floor

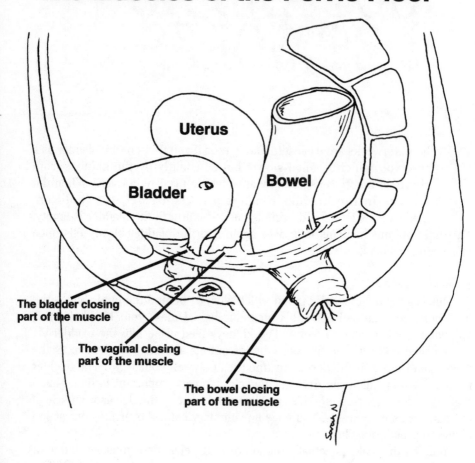

Uterus

Bladder

Bowel

The bladder closing
part of the muscle

The vaginal closing
part of the muscle

The bowel closing
part of the muscle

obvious goal: it fires off a reflex which travels from the pelvic floor back to the bladder and tells the detrusor muscles to stop contracting and pushing out urine. As the sphincter and pelvic floor muscles relax, another reflex fires, this time telling the detrusor to contract. In other words, the urethral sphincter and pelvic floor muscles tell the bladder muscles when to pump and when to relax and quietly fill up again.

Summary

As the bladder fills, nerve endings in the wall of the bladder tell you when you are getting close to full (let's say about 350mls). You hold on until it suits you to go, then, when you are ready:
• the muscles of the pelvic floor and urethral sphincter relax,
• the bladder detrusor muscle contracts until all the urine is passed,
• the pelvic floor contracts and the outlet is closed.

So you can see just how much the pelvic floor really is in charge of your waterworks. It acts as the conductor of the symphony of stopping and starting. It controls the filling and emptying sequences of the bladder. Can you see what might happen if these pelvic floor muscles lost some of their strength? Can you see how the pelvic floor might lose control over the bladder and the bladder might begin to contract whenever it wanted to, not when you wanted it to? This is called urgency – sometimes described as a "knee-crossing, eye-watering desire to pee". Urgency occurs when the bladder begins to take charge of stopping and starting the orchestra. It's a hard taskmaster – a bossy tyrant that can rule your life. When your bladder is in charge, as soon as you wake in the morning your mind begins to plan your daily activities. These all centre around your urgency. You need to 'go' as soon as the urge hits you. Even a simple shopping trip has to be planned to the last detail – where are the toilets? How far between them? Will I make it all the way in the bus? After a few years of living like this, it's no wonder some women become 'bladder hermits', confining themselves to their homes because they feel safe. Their so-called 'little secret' now dominates their lives.

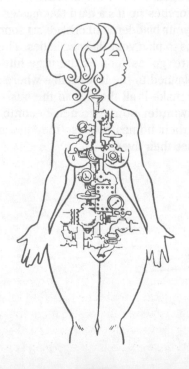

CHAPTER 3

THE MULTIFUNCTIONAL PELVIC FLOOR

There are a number of things that can cause women to lose control of their waterworks. If you have an understanding of how this happens, it's easier for you to help yourself over the hurdles along the road to recovery. Losing control is most often the fault of weak pelvic floor muscles, the multi-functional muscles which form the floor of the pelvic basin. The pelvic floor muscles are made up of two distinct types of muscle fibres. One type (slow twitch, type II muscle fibre) is designed to hold on for lengthy periods, just like calf muscles which help you to stand for a long time. Slow twitch muscle fibres help support the abdominal organs and also work constantly to keep urine up inside the bladder until a suitable time and place for urination is found. Few of us are aware of this muscle activity, it tends to regulate itself and is something we take for granted. The other type of muscle fibres in the pelvic floor (fast twitch, type I) are designed to act strongly and quickly, but do not hold on for long periods. Fast twitch muscle fibres act as an extra closing force during a laugh, cough or sneeze. An extra squeeze is needed when you lift heavy objects or whenever you have to 'hold on' for any reason, for example there is no toilet available or you're about to clinch a big deal over lunch, having had one or two glasses of wine.

This extra squeeze to prevent a leak is called 'the knack'. This is one knack you really need to get hold of. Remember, it's this extra closing force that stops the bladder muscle, the detrusor, from contracting as well. It puts you in control. It's easy to understand the action of these different types of muscle fibres if you look at the calf muscles once again. Compare the slow twitch standing/walking action to the fast twitch of jumping or running when the calf muscle come into play in a totally different way. So you can see how one single group of muscles can do quite different jobs in a very efficient manner. If one group of fibres is more efficient than the other, then obviously one job will be done better than the other, but usually the muscles of the pelvic floor suffer equally and both areas work less efficiently if anything is wrong.

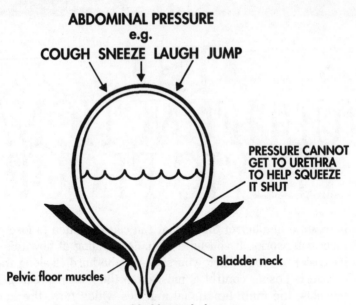

ABDOMINAL PRESSURE
e.g.
COUGH SNEEZE LAUGH JUMP

PRESSURE CANNOT
GET TO URETHRA
TO HELP SQUEEZE
IT SHUT

Bladder neck

Pelvic floor muscles

Poor support – bladder neck descent
URINE ESCAPES

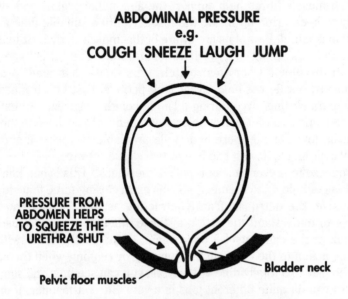

ABDOMINAL PRESSURE
e.g.
COUGH SNEEZE LAUGH JUMP

PRESSURE FROM
ABDOMEN HELPS
TO SQUEEZE THE
URETHRA SHUT

Bladder neck

Pelvic floor muscles

'Good support – no bladder neck descent
NO URINE ESCAPES

Generally speaking, it's impossible to separate the different muscles of the pelvic floor and almost impossible to contract them individually: they were designed to work as a complete unit. In doing this they fulfil many roles, not just that of keeping you dry, although this is probably the job you are most aware of. However, we need to take a closer look at how the pelvic floor muscles function overall, to look at all the different jobs these muscles do. You will not only be surprised, but you will also realise just how the pelvic floor is letting you down in more ways than one.

Getting A Grip On Your Man ... Sexual Response

The most important muscle of the pelvic floor is the Pubococcygeus (PC). The PC is one of the deeper layers of the pelvic floor muscles. While the PC has sometimes been called the "love muscle", it is the more superficial layer of the pelvic floor muscles that have a specific sexual function. These smaller muscles (called bulbo-spongiosis and ischi-ocavernosus) are responsible for pumping blood to the clitoris in women (and the penis in men), so that it becomes full and erect during arousal. Another function of these muscles is rhythmic contraction at orgasm. In theory, women should be able to improve their level of arousal by the rhythmic contraction of these pelvic floor muscles.

Apart from the superficial pelvic floor muscles, women with strong PC muscles probably enjoy the bonus of good sexual sensation. The pelvic floor muscles are directly responsible for the amount of sensation that women feel during intercourse. The PC wraps around the outer one third of the vagina which corresponds to that part of the vagina generally known as the orgasmic platform The PC also directly affects the amount of sexual sensation male partners feel. In other words, the PC muscles help you to get a firm grip on your man.

Believe it or not, the lining of the vagina is not well endowed with sensory nerve endings and really does not have a lot of sensation. If you place your index finger in your vagina and gently draw your fingernail down the inside surface, you will find that you feel almost nothing. In fact, vaginal sensations come mostly from the pelvic floor muscles that loop around behind the vagina. All muscles have nerve endings within them which respond positively to stretch. The stronger and firmer the muscle, the more of these nerve endings it contains. Therefore a strong, firm PC will be stretched by the erect penis. As the glans (tip) of the penis moves back and forth during intercourse, these firm muscles will rhythmically stretch and relax, thus heightening vaginal sensations. Your ability to achieve orgasm might be boosted as pelvic floor muscle strength increases. All in all, you can see that sexually speaking, these muscles play a vital role. So, when you have a strong PC muscle, then the sky is really the limit sexually.

Holding up (or Falling Down) On The Job

The pelvic floor muscles actually form the floor of the pelvic basin (that's how they get their name) and act as a safety net for all the organs that sit low in the abdomen or within the bony pelvis. When the pelvic floor falls down on the job, two things can happen:

Stress Incontinence: firstly, those forces which normally press on the urethra to keep the floodgates closed, now actually help to open the floodgates, thus you are presented with the problem of Stress Incontinence. This form of incontinence occurs every time pressure (stress) is exerted on the bladder, eg running, jumping, coughing, laughing, lifting or sneezing. This is the most common form of incontinence and during urine loss of this type, the bladder muscle itself remains inactive.

Bowel Control

One very important role played by the muscles of the pelvic floor is that of normal bowel control. The pelvic floor muscles not only support the bowel and help us to actually 'hear the call of nature', but they are directly responsible for giving you confident bowel control. Strong and efficient pelvic floor muscles allow you to feel the sensation that you 'need to go'. Another part of the muscle allows you to 'hold on' until you are ready to go. When the time comes to open your bowels, a healthy pelvic floor muscle actually helps to hold the anus in the proper position that allows it to open as the bowel is emptied. Poor pelvic floor muscle function can aggravate or cause constipation. It can also lead to leaking from the back passage. For more information about bowel function and the pelvic floor muscles see "Let's Get Things Moving" by Chiarelli and Markwell, another book in this series published by Health Books.

Prolapse

When the pelvic organs drop down (and sometimes through) the pelvic diaphragm, the result is prolapse. Most women have heard this term before – prolapse is an extremely common complaint and is not only caused by weak pelvic floor muscles, but also by over-stretching the ligaments that normally support the abdominal organs.

Pelvic organ prolapse is very common. When older women were asked if they had ever been told by a doctor that they had a prolapse, almost one quarter of them answered yes. Significant numbers of women who leak urine also have pelvic organ prolapse of one sort or another.

Women often describe these prolapses as "a cherry just sitting at the opening down there". Most often noticed for the first time in the shower, these protrusions tend to occur when there have been higher than usual levels of physical activity. Prolapses are usually symptom-free, but can cause back pain with dragging sensations in the abdomen. The most common form of prolapse is cystocoele when the bladder presses down into the vagina. If the bladder drops, because the tissues that suspend and support it have been over-stretched, then any pressures from within the abdomen (eg when you cough, laugh, lift or sneeze) can actually cause urine to leak out.

There are three types of pelvic organ prolapse, which may occur singularly, or you may suffer from all three.

Uterine prolapse generally appears following childbirth where the strains of labour can cause over-stretching of the ligaments which support the uterus. The pelvic floor offers little support immediately following the birth of a baby and the general level of physical exhaustion associated with caring for a new baby (the night feedings and the mountains of washing) do nothing to help the situation. Bladder prolapse occurs when the bladder sags into the vagina.

When women have a prolapsed rectum, they often complain not so much of constipation, but that they have great difficulty actually getting the faeces out of the body. There may be a sensation of incomplete evacuation of the bowel. They push and push – to no avail – but pushing actually aggravates the prolapse. The very simple and effective solution to this problem is to press up the whole area in front of the rectum with the hand, or by inserting two fingers into the vagina and gently pressing backwards towards the tailbone.

Women are commonly advised to have prolapses surgically repaired. There is no real indication that this is necessary at all unless the prolapse is causing discomfort such as abdominal or low back pain, a dragging sensation low in the abdomen, painful intercourse, the feeling that there is not enough room in the vagina to accommodate your partner's penis or problems associated with using your bladder or bowels. You should be able to decide for yourself whether the symptoms warrant surgery or not. You are in control of the situation, you should make the decision. The pelvic floor exercises described later in this book have limited value in the treatment of prolapse, but they may help in two ways:

1. If the safety net is strengthened, the prolapse might not become any worse.

2. During breastfeeding, uterine prolapse can be aggravated by the lack of circulating hormones that normally help the pelvic floor muscles to work properly. Therefore constant watch must be kept over the pelvic floor muscles at this time.

Working As A Guide

Finally, the pelvic floor muscles act as a guide during delivery of your baby and are responsible for turning and guiding the baby's head as it moves down through the birth canal and into the outside world.

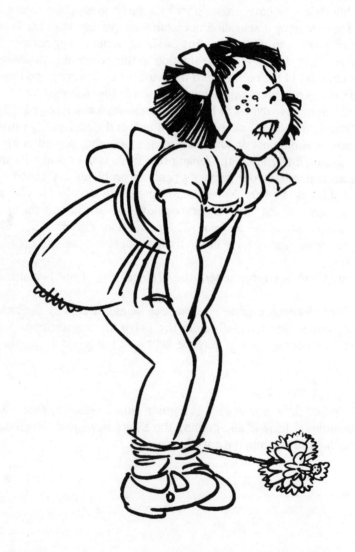

CHAPTER 4

THE RISE AND FALL OF THE PELVIC FLOOR

You've all seen the little girl ... she is using deferment techniques. These techniques are designed help you hold on. They include:
- pelvic floor contractions (if she knows how),
- pressure on her perineum,
- her mind is elsewhere,
- her mouth is puckering tightly.

Even though you may not have had much bladder control as a child, it doesn't mean you can't take control now. Being able to contract the muscles of the pelvic floor is something that women learn to do, they are not born with the ability to use these muscles. Some women never gain control of the basic mechanism. Learning control is easy – you might just need a little understanding and guidance. If your pelvic floor muscles need retraining, you will probably find it easier if you can understand all those things that might have contributed to this weakness. It may have been caused by one single event, but usually it's a combination of factors that bring about the downfall of the pelvic floor muscles.

Did It Rise?

Most important of all, did your pelvic floor rise in the first place? Have you ever had control of your pelvic floor muscles? More than one in ten women who have never had a baby leak urine at times. Many young girls have poor control of the pelvic floor muscles because their urinating patterns do nothing to encourage the pelvic muscles to hold on. To begin, little girls are encouraged to 'wee' according to when Mum wants them to, not when they need to. Remember your mother saying, "Go to the toilet now, dear, we're going in the car to Gran's."? On arrival, it was, "Go to the toilet, we're going to have dinner now". Immediately after dinner: "Go to the toilet, dear, we're going

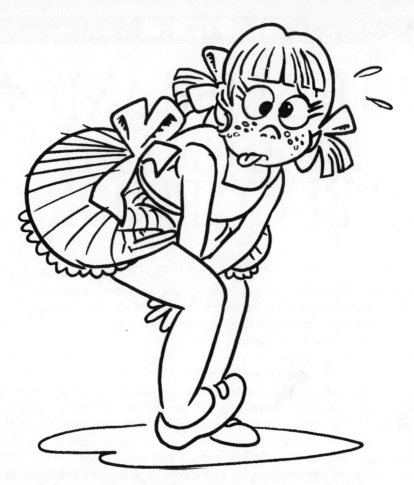

home now". As soon as you arrive home: "Do a wee now, dear, it's time to go to bed". Little boys get no such encouragement. Why? Because they can urinate just about anywhere: if the need arises, little boys can manage to 'go', using Mum, a handy bush or telegraph pole to hide behind. Not so little girls. They are often actively encouraged into frequency – encouraged into "doing a wee just in case". This is perhaps one of the greatest wrongs a mother can do her daughter. Girls should be encouraged to urinate only when they need to. They have the ability to hold on until a suitable place can be found; they could probably hold on longer that Mum if the truth be known.

By encouraging young girls to hold on, mothers help them to develop pelvic floor control. It's a fallacy that 'holding on' for a long time will cause urinary problems – this is just not so. The only time a woman should not be encouraged to hold on is when she is suffering from some form of cystitis. It's also interesting to note that in some less developed countries, young women are taught pelvic floor contractions by the midwives as part of their adult initiation ceremonies. While boys are circumcised or pass through other rituals, the girls learn to contract their vaginas around the examining fingers of the midwife. In various cultures women are not allowed to resume sexual relationships with their husbands following the birth of their children until they can once again contract the pelvic floor muscles around the palpating fingers of the midwife.

Another socially contributing factor is that many women in these countries adopt the squatting position as the most comfortable way to sit. The pelvic floor muscles have to work strongly in this position to prevent leaking and because these women squat to carry out many of their daily activities, the muscles become extremely strong.

Did It Fall Or Was It Pushed?

The graph on page 25 illustrates the percentage of women who suffer urine loss during the daytime. It shows their average ages and gives an indication of what might have started the leakage. To understand more fully, each factor will be looked at individually starting with those factors which can cause pelvic floor muscle weakness.

Pregnancy

About 65 per cent of women complain of incontinence during pregnancy. Incontinence during pregnancy can begin in the first, second or third trimester. While women experience either stress incontinence or urge incontinence during pregnancy, most women complain of 'mixed' incontinence – they have stress leaks which occur together with a sense of urgency at times.

The cause of the incontinence experienced during pregnancy is not really clear, but hormones are thought to play an important role. The hormones work to soften the outlet of the uterus (cervix) to allow the baby's head to emerge. At the same time, other supporting structures are thought to undergo the same 'softening process'. The weight of the baby itself is then pressing upon support structures that do not have the same tensile strength during pregnancy that they normally have. Women who leak urine during pregnancy have been shown to have less support around the bladder neck, and it is not sure at what point in time (if ever) following delivery that the bladder neck support returns to normal.

Frequency and nocturia during pregnancy can be caused by a number of things. Firstly, women take in a lot more fluid during pregnancy to provide the fluid required within the sac around the baby as well as the blood supply of the baby itself. Pressure of the baby makes it difficult for fluid in the legs to circulate freely. Only at night when the pregnant woman lies in bed with her legs up, does the fluid have a chance to move up into the kidneys. This explains why many pregnant women get up frequently throughout the night to urinate.

Labour and Delivery

The next important cause of incontinence is vaginal delivery. Almost forty per cent of women who have had four babies or more with a vaginal birth, complain of urinary stress incontinence, with each delivery further damaging the pelvic floor muscles. This is the result of a combination of factors, best understood by looking at each in turn.

Anatomical: The average birth size of babies today is much bigger than in earlier generations. This is because of the high standard of prenatal care and because nutritional advice for pregnant women is much more accessible, as is the availability of a well-balanced diet.

Mechanical: As the baby's head moves through the birth canal to the outside world, forces acting on the bladder, urethra and most especially the pelvic floor muscles and all its supports, can damage these structures. Tearing or simple overstretching of the muscles, ligaments, connective tissues and their nerve supply cause progressive weakness with each baby in turn. Women with babies delivered by forceps, by ventouse (suction cup) or birthing babies heavier than 4000g (four kilograms) are thought to be more at risk for developing urinary incontinence at a later stage. Deliveries such as these have a tendency to lead to slightly more pelvic floor nerve damage.

Hormonal: It takes anything up to six weeks for circulating relaxin levels to disappear after the birth of a baby. This means that the muscles of the pelvic floor cannot return to their fullest potential strength until that time. Breastfeeding mothers can have very low levels of the hormone oestrogen. Some nerve junctions in the bladder base and urethra sphincter require oestrogen to function properly, so breastfeeding women need to pay special attention to pelvic floor exercises even though they may see little improvement for their effort. These exercises will encourage those muscle fibres which can work to do so and, as soon as oestrogen levels become normal again, so should the tone in the supporting structures of the bladder. Oestrogen levels rise when ovulation begins again, that is, just before menstruation returns. It is also important for breastfeeding women to realise that they have very low volumes of urine. Much of the fluid taken into the body is used to produce breast milk therefore less may be filtered out into the bladder.

Any breastfeeding women who is experiencing urinary stress incontinence should take special note: there is very little urine in your bladder – your pelvic floor muscles should be able to keep you dry. If not, you need to seek help immediately. For a breastfeeding mother to be leaking urine means that her urinary control is very poor and in need of urgent attention.

Neurological: It's important to remember that the pelvic floor contracts reflexively before we cough or sneeze. This is a protective reflex against leaking which works via the nervous system. Think back to immediately after the birth of your baby: you will recall just how sore your bottom felt, like sitting on a bed of nails. You thought things would never be the same again and you

INCIDENCE OF INCONTINENCE AT VARIOUS AGES IN EACH SEX

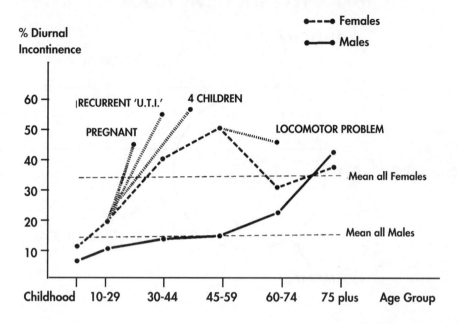

● - - ● Females
●———● Males

% Diurnal Incontinence

RECURRENT 'U.T.I.' 4 CHILDREN

PREGNANT LOCOMOTOR PROBLEM

Mean all Females

Mean all Males

Childhood 10-29 30-44 45-59 60-74 75 plus Age Group

R.M. MILLARD 1986

were probably right. This is when you may have lost, or given up, conscious control over the muscles of your pelvic floor. If you looked at your perineum at this stage you probably didn't recognise that swollen black and blue area between your legs. You probably laughed at any suggestion made by a nurse or a physiotherapist that you "try to pull up the area between your legs". You treated your pelvic floor very gingerly. Using your bowels was a nightmare, getting your stitches to heal nicely and keeping yourself clean and dry was about all you could cope with. Squeeze up tight? They had to be kidding! Called 'reflex inhibition', this is a well-known condition that physiotherapists see all the time after surgery on, or following damage to, any joint – especially the knee or ankle. Reflex inhibition is the brain's way of protecting those areas of the body which are damaged, swollen and painful. Unless these reflexes are re-established, chronic injury results.

Most people realise that if an ankle is sprained badly, there is a permanent tendency for that ankle to twist and give way again. When treating sporting injuries such as these, the physiotherapist concentrates on re-training the protective reflex action of the muscles around the ankle. There is no point in treating the joint without re-training the reflex, the injured player will be back within weeks complaining of the same problem. And so it is with pelvic floor

THE MANY FORCES OF LABOUR & DELIVERY THAT AFFECT THE PELVIC FLOOR

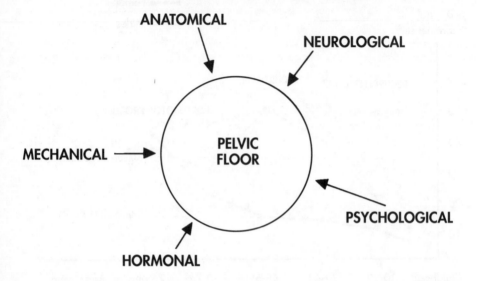

following childbirth. The protective reflex contraction of the pelvic floor when you cough or sneeze is lost, never to return. This protective reflex can be re-learned. You can teach yourself to actively squeeze and lift before each cough or sneeze. This 'leak stopping' squeeze and lift has been given the name of 'the knack'. Getting the knack after a delivery is extremely important.

Another neurological factor contributing to incontinence after vaginal delivery has been mentioned before. This is actual damage to the nerves which supply the muscles of the pelvic floor caused when forceps are used, or when the woman has a second stage lasting longer than one hour, especially with a heavy baby. Second stage is generally considered to be that point in the labour when the baby's head is out of the uterus and sitting on the perineum. Usually this is the stage where you desperately want to push. This nerve damage is not always apparent immediately following the birth. The extra burden placed on the nerve damaged pelvic floor by years of pushing and straining in women who suffer from constipation, in women who are overweight, who have a chronic cough or do repeated heavy lifting, in the long term eventually leads to leaking urine.

Psychological: Childbirth is a time of great upheaval in a woman's life. Thoughts crowding for attention along with the new baby include its siblings, its new dad, and the responsibilities of caring for what has been described as a "crying alimentary canal" that needs feeding at one end and cleaning at the other. There is little time to worry whether the pelvic muscles are working properly. Most women are very aware of the ravages of pregnancy and childbirth: weight gain, loss of muscle tone (especially in the tummy) and a general lowering of endurance levels.

Many women take a very positive approach to these body changes and set about exercising to get back their 'pre-pregnant' figure. But the pelvic floor is unseen and forgotten ... until it makes its presence felt as a damp spot. By this time, some years may have passed although it can happen immediately after the baby is born. This is also when you realise that your sexual response is not what it used to be. This post-natal loss of libido is easily put down to the rigours of caring for a new baby, post-natal blues. It's often, however, quite a different thing: the PC muscle has lost its grip. Your ability to be aroused returns, but you never seen to get enough stimulation to reach orgasm. The woman who masturbates to orgasm might feel that reaching her peak takes longer.

All in all, the pelvic floor muscles tend to get ignored after childbirth: out of sight, out of mind. Childbirth educators sometimes place greater emphasis on re-training abdominal muscle strength during the birth than on strengthening pelvic floor contractions. Even if you do not suffer post-natal urinary stress incontinence, your pelvic floor muscles have taken a real beating during the birth and a self-organised, post-natal exercise routine should be started within 24 hours of the baby's delivery.

Physical: The pelvic floor muscles suffer from general fatigue, just as all muscles in the body do. A new mother works long hours and has an increased load of work. It is important to realise that fatigue is yet another causative factor in the post-natal fall of the pelvic floor. Resting with the feet up is scoffed at by most new mothers – who has the time? But what a price to pay later for ignoring this simple fact. One simple reason for women not doing pelvic floor exercises is just remembering them. It's certainly worth considering some reminder or other, stuck up on the fridge, the back of the toilet door or on the wall above the baby's change table. A simple message such "HAVE YOU DONE YOURS TODAY?" might be all you need.

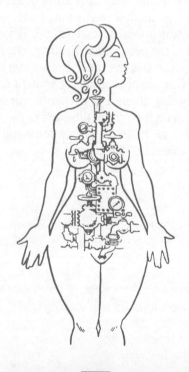

CHAPTER 5

NOT ONLY, BUT ALSO'

When women experience incontinence it's not always weakness of the pelvic floor that has thrown the spanner in the works. This chapter looks at other factors that can lead to problems with the waterworks. Look again at the graph on Page 25 and you will notice that cystitis, childhood bedwetting, ageing and mobility problems have yet to be explained.

Cystitis: Recurrent Urinary Tract Infections

The number of women who suffer recurrent cystitis is astounding. In medical terms, "cyst" means "bladder", while "itis" on the end of any word means "inflammation of", hence cystitis simply means any inflammation of the bladder. While inflammation always accompanies infection, the reverse is not true: it is possible to suffer inflammation of the bladder without any infection. Cystitis commonly manifests itself as an urgent desire to urinate, however, when you reach the toilet, you pass only a tiny amount accompanied by an almost unendurable pain. This is coupled with frequency (every 10 or 20 minutes the burning desire returns) and maybe a dull pain low in the abdomen.

In many instances, these symptoms do signify an infection, especially if there is a rise in body temperature with chills and fever: you will need to visit your doctor for a pathology test and take a full course of antibiotics if infection is present. Many women with recurrent attacks of cystitis know that the antibiotics usually prescribed for the complaint sometimes have absolutely no effect on their signs and symptoms. This is because the inflammation may be caused by an undiagnosed allergic reaction and many of these women will respond to the simple strategies used to fight all allergies. Some of the women who suffer the discomfort of recurrent cystitis will later develop the signs and symptoms of bladder instability. This is also true for those women who suffer what is commonly called "the urethral syndrome" or "non-specific urethritis". Both these terms describe the inflammation of the urethra that often follows cystitis or an infection within the urethra. It usually begins within an infection with the bladder or the urethra. This infection often responds well to a course of antibiotics, but the inflammation that always goes hand-in-hand with the infection does not respond to these medications.

To understand this very common problem, it is important to know what is happening within the bladder and the urethra, giving extra thought to those rather complicated reflexes mentioned earlier. The bladder lining becomes inflamed either from the infection, an allergic reaction or from tissue damage caused mechanically. As with the tissues that are inflamed, the mucosal lining of the bladder becomes red, hot and swollen. Obviously, if urine comes in contact with this red, swollen bladder lining the result will be felt as a burning, stinging pain. When the urine is "stronger" than usual – as it almost always is with an infection – these unpleasant symptoms are worse. This explains the awful sensations and the frequency that go with cystitis. The bladder is saying, "Help! Get this urine out! It is stinging me and burning my insides!" But what about the urgency? The urgency that goes with cystitis really has to be felt to be believed. This is where the reflexes come into play. Let's look again at all the mechanisms involved in completely emptying the bladder.

1. As you sit on the toilet, the pelvic floor muscles relax.

2. A reflex is fired that tells the bladder muscle (the detrusor) to start contracting. This pushes the urine out of the bladder.

3. As the urine moves into the outlet tube (urethra), another reflex fires off. This reflex keeps the bladder muscle contracting until all the urine has been passed. When no more urine is passing into the urethra, the reflex tells the bladder to stop contracting.

4. The pelvic floor muscles contract to squeeze the urethra shut. This also works to stop the bladder contraction.

So, what goes wrong? Look at part two of the explanation above. When the base of the bladder and the urethra are inflamed, the reflexes in those areas start working overtime, forcing you to go now even though it is only 10 minutes, or less, since you last went. The urine is burning the inflamed area and this is causing the bladder to contract again and again. An inflammatory reaction can also be caused by tissue damaged by mechanical means. For instance, honeymoon cystitis is caused by the thrusting of the penis against the urethra and/or the bladder base. Such damage can also be caused by wearing a tampon incorrectly: if it is too large for your vagina, or if it twists sideways, then bruising of the urethra can follow. Bruising is also accompanied by localised inflammation.

Causes of Cystitis or the "Urethral Syndrome"

• Infection travelling directly from the vagina or the anus. Sometimes carried by the bloodstream from other parts of the body.

• An allergic reaction to some foods, bath additives or talcum powder.

• Honeymoon cystitis or traumatic urethritis caused by other factors eg ill-fitting tampons, vigorous masturbation, horse-riding or uncomfortable bicycle seats.

• Any irritation of the external genital area from a vaginal infection of any kind. The infection need not travel up to the bladder, the inflammation just might, however.

• General body fatigue – if you are tired and run down, so are your body's defence systems.

Pelvic floor muscle weakness:
a) The resting tone of the pelvic floor muscles needs to be high enough to help the sphincter keep the urethra tightly shut against invading germs.
b) If the pelvic floor muscles are not supporting the local tissues properly, the blood supply to these tissues will not be as good as it should be. A healthy blood supply is the tissues' first line of defence against any infection or inflammation.

Low oestrogen states:
The urethra, vagina and bladder neck are rich in oestrogen receptors. At times when oestrogen levels fall below normal, these particular tissues lose their rich blood supply and suffer a condition called atrophy. Atrophy occurs most commonly following menopause but can also occur following surgical removal of both ovaries or while a mother is breastfeeding

Simple Strategies
Beware! Recurrent cystitis might be concealing other, more serious bladder conditions. If the simple measures that follow do not seem to be helping your signs and symptoms, please see your doctor for a thorough examination of both your urine and your urinary tract.
Try these steps at the first sign of any irritation:
• Drink as much water as you can manage. This will help to dilute your urine.
• Drink one small bottle of cranberry juice each day. This ancient remedy has been shown to be very effective against many forms of bladder infection. The juice should be taken each day and many women drink it to prevent as well as to treat cystitis.
• Take a urinary alkaliniser eg one rounded teaspoon of bicarbonate of soda, or go to your pharmacist for his/her recommendation. Keep some alkiniser on hand at all times.
• This is the only time, ever, that you should not 'hold on'. Go when your bladder tells you.
• Put your feet up and relax for 2 or 3 hours.
• Avoid drinking coffee, strong tea or alcohol.
• Avoid intercourse or using tampons until all signs and symptoms have subsided. See chapter 10, "Prevention is Better Than Cure", for hints to avoid this painful complaint.
• If your cystitis is associated with intercourse, try to urinate following intercourse each time.
• If postmenopausal, the oestrogen found in plants (phyto-oestrogens) might be of some help. Soymilk has been shown to be high in phyto-oestrogens as have linseed and soy beans themselves.

• Have your bladder checked to see if you are emptying properly. Residual urine can lead to problems with infections (see later under Testing - ultrasound)

Menopause

Many women sail through life blissfully unaware of the time bomb ticking away between their legs. They are totally unaware of all the stresses and strains that have weakened their pelvic floor muscles. That is, until they pass through the menopause which is often 'the straw that breaks the camel's back'. Just how this comes about is quite simple to understand. There are special receptors within the bladder base and the urethra which need oestrogen to function properly. During menopause, this oestrogen level drops off rather dramatically. Remember, at this stage we are adding insult to injury – the injury as already described in the previous chapter generally occurs with pregnancy or childbirth.

The oestrogen factor is also responsible for the thinning effect that can occur within the vagina and urethra. These linings are very similar in design and construction and they each react in the same way to the lack of oestrogen that accompanies menopause. Any post-menopausal woman who suffers vaginal atrophy also suffers atrophy of the urethral lining. Atrophic vaginitis causes dryness, itching and/or pain with red, sometimes bleeding, patches on the skin around the labia and within the vagina. The vagina loses its 'padding' inside, and there is a loss of sexual lubrication. The vaginal opening can become narrowed, the vaginal walls bleed easily and can react strongly to even the most gentle artificial lubricants by stinging and burning. Intercourse can be very painful.

Surgical menopause can be just as difficult to cope with as natural menopause. When a woman has had her ovaries removed, for whatever reason, unless hormone replacement therapy is started she will, in effect, go through the menopause. Surgical castration or Oophorectomy is the term used to describe the removal of both ovaries from a woman's body. This often accompanies a hysterectomy, which is the surgical removal of the uterus. Sometimes loss of bladder control might follow a hysterectomy even if there was complete control before the surgery. A sad state of affairs that need not occur if there is hormonal replacement treatment, which maintains hormone levels at a pre-hysterectomy level.

Ageing

All muscles over which we have control tend to decrease in bulk and strength as part of the natural ageing process. This is not inevitable and can be helped. A simple exercise program given to elderly women may give them back their dignity and enable them to live life to the fullest. Another problem that often goes hand-in-hand with ageing is the loss of mobility. For many elderly women, incontinence begins with their inability to make it to the toilet in time because of arthritis. Coupled with this lack of mobility is a decrease in

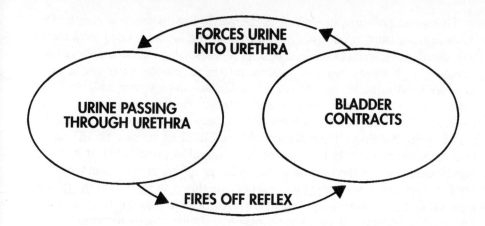

FORCES URINE INTO URETHRA

URINE PASSING THROUGH URETHRA

BLADDER CONTRACTS

FIRES OFF REFLEX

reaction time – a decrease in the time between the bladder message saying "I need to be emptied" and the actual bladder contraction which starts the emptying process. If stiff, arthritic knees and ankles mean a slow trip to the toilet, then accidents are more likely to happen. Any increase in the weight of the abdominal organs is going to increase the load on the pelvic floor. If you increase the pressures pushing down on an already weakened pelvic floor, then more urine loss is bound to happen.

It's a fact of life that many women suffer weight increase following the menopause (surgical or natural). The muscles of the pelvic floor have enough of a job keeping up as hormone levels fall without the added burden of extra weight. Every time you cough, sneeze or laugh the extra weight you are carrying pushes down on your pelvic floor, stretching it more and more, weakening it yet further. An increase in weight on top of the menopause is bad enough, but if you add the problems of constipation or chronic cough, then it's 'Goodbye Charlie' – your pelvic floor doesn't stand a chance of being able to cope.

Apart from the muscles of the pelvic floor ageing, the bladder muscle itself can lose some of its power. This leads to incomplete emptying of the bladder and residual urine. Any residual urine left in the bladder after urination has taken place has a tendency to become infected. For this as well as other reasons, a doctor or continence adviser should manage a problem with residual urine.

Constipation and/or Chronic Cough

When a woman suffers chronic constipation, she spends time every day attacking the pelvic floor muscles, making them weaker and weaker. Pushing and straining against a set of muscles that are usually already in a very weakened state does further damage. Every time she strains at stool (the term used to describe this action) the bulging, downward pressure acts on the whole of the pelvic floor causing even further stretching and damage.

This same pressure is applied to the pelvic floor when you cough. The downward pressure is not usually as strong as the pressure used for a bowel movement, but it tends to be done dozens of times a day – each and every time you cough. Smokers beware, asthma suffers take note: your pelvic floor muscles need to be stronger than normal to counteract your coughing. It's never too late to increase the strength of the pelvic floor muscles. So if you have a chronic cough, for whatever reason, very special attention should be paid to your 'holding on' mechanism. It's not unusual to hear about elderly women becoming totally incontinent after a bout of pneumonia. It isn't the infection that causes the incontinence, it's the coughing plus the fact that they are generally in bed for some time and become slower in their movements and confused. The women's pelvic floor strength is lost by the constant unaccustomed strain of coughing – never to return unless someone shows them how. Women should support their perineum if they suffer any pelvic floor weakness along with any complaint that causes coughing. Simply 'holding on' with firm hand pressure over the perineum can save this area from damage by not allowing it to over-stretch with every cough.

Being Overweight

Studies show that the number of women who leak urine increases with their bodymass. Every kilo that you are carrying over and above what would be the normal bodymass for you is placing an extra load on the structures of the pelvic floor – the muscles, as well as the connective, supporting tissue. It may not be necessary for you to lose much weight at all in order to notice a difference in the number of times or the amount of leaking you experience.

Drugs

Drugs do not really have a big role to play in the management of urinary incontinence. In fact, in the elderly, they can actually cause a whole lot of problems. Some drugs commonly prescribed for high blood pressure (hypertension) actually lead to lower function levels of the mechanisms that work to promote continence. One popular blood pressure drug is Minipress (Prazosin). This drug actually stops nerve endings – the same ones that are affected by estrogen levels – from transmitting messages to the bladder and urethral sphincters. Fluid tablets, taken to eliminate excess fluid from the body, are frequently prescribed with medication for high blood pressure and/or heart problems. Elderly people often take them too early in the morning before they have their joints moving properly and this can cause accidents. Check with a doctor and see if they might be taken at lunch-time. Some arthritis tablets (Surgam) have been found to lead to urgency and frequency in some people.

You must accept that any chemical substance which affects normal body function is a drug. With this in mind the effects of caffeine and alcohol must be understood. Caffeine is found in coffee and cola beverages and to a lesser extent in tea. Percolated coffee contains much more caffeine than instant coffee. Different drugs, naturally, have different actions and while caffeine does not affect the bladder support system like Prazosin, it is just as troublesome. It irritates the bladder muscle itself and helps to cause frequency and urgency. Alcohol has yet another effect on the waterworks. Alcohol is a diuretic which means that it pulls water out of the body tissues where it is stored and pushes this water out through the kidneys and into the bladder. When you drink alcohol you tend to pass a higher volume of fluid than you take in. Alcohol also tends to decrease the ability to co-ordinate the complicated act of 'holding on'.

Imagine this scene: You're out to dinner. It's a celebration and throughout the evening you manage to consume an entire bottle of wine. The meal is finished with a few cups of very strong, black coffee and perhaps a liqueur or port. It's a cold night and as you journey home, every traffic light seems to be red. By the time you turn the corner of your street you are absolutely busting to go to the toilet. The taxi stops and you pay the driver quickly and tumble out. You walk rapidly to the door, fumbling in your bag for the key. Your plight is desperate. You know you are going to lose everything in a minute if the door doesn't open. Success, it opens. You hurry down the hall. Relief is near. By the time you enter the bathroom, the water is escaping, running uncontrollably down your legs.

This is quite a common scene caused by both the caffeine and the alcohol. The alcohol draws the water out of the body's storage area and also clouds your awareness which makes it hard to recognise the normal body signals. These signals tend to be noticed much later than usual, giving you much less time to respond when your bladder says, "empty me soon". On top of all this, the caffeine irritates the bladder, in effect saying to your bladder, "okay, contract now". You are, I know, familiar with this scene. In most cases women blame the alcohol, but take it from me, the coffee plays quite a major role.

Spinal Problems

Pelvic floor weakness can sometimes occur when spinal nerves are damaged. This can happen if you suffer disc problems or other joint dysfunction in the lower lumbar spine. The nerves that carry the message to your pelvic floor muscles do not function properly and varying levels of pelvic floor paralysis can occur.

Other Factors

There are many causes that lead to problems with the waterworks. These include catheters, brain damage such as a stroke, Parkinson's Disease and diabetes. One particular problem area is bedwetting with many bed-wetters developing problems with their waterworks later in life. These problems generally fall into the category of 'an unstable bladder' and treatment is directed along the lines of the bladder retaining program explained in chapter 7.

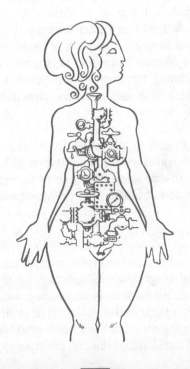

CHAPTER 6

TESTING, TESTING

Most women with waterworks problems will find they respond to the simple self-help instructions given in the next chapter. If any doubt exists in your mind, check with your doctor first. The following procedures have been described so that you might understand some of the many things that might already have been done for you or tests that your own doctor might suggest.

Urinalysis: The inevitable specimen. The urine is sent to a pathology laboratory to be checked for a number of things including the presence of blood, infections, diabetes, abnormal cells and protein.

X-ray: This can show any spinal problems, kidney stones or bladder stones. Your bowel can be seen in an X-ray as well as your pelvis, sacroiliac joint and symphysis pubis (where the public bones meet).

Cystoscopy: Here the surgeon uses a tiny instrument passed up the urethra. The doctor can now see inside the bladder. He/she cannot see the bladder or sphincter functioning – all he/she can see is the lining of the bladder itself. The surgeon can check to see that there are no areas of inflammation, no growths (polyps), stones or tumours and can take cells samples from the wall of the bladder to have them checked by a pathologist.

Ultrasound: This is a non-invasive way of showing an image of the bladder and is much like the ultrasound used during pregnancy to scan the baby within the uterus. You will be asked to attend for an ultrasound with a full bladder. The ultrasound image can show up a bladder neck that is not closing properly, as well as showing leaking during a cough. After you empty your bladder, an ultrasound image can show if there is any urine left in the bladder. This is called residual urine. If you have residual urine it means that your bladder is not emptying properly. There is always a bit of urine left within the bladder, but this should never be more than 50mls in a healthy, young to middle-aged person. As we age, we tend to have a higher urinary residual than this. High urinary residuals can lead to recurrent bladder infections and in elderly people, a bladder that is not emptying well can cause all sorts of problems including a condition called overflow incontinence.

Urodynamic Investigation: This is really the 'Rolls-Royce' of examinations. The doctor can see the bladder at work and watch the dynamic parts of 'holding on' and gushing out. Because abnormalities can be seen as they happen so, often, can the reasons behind them. This examination shows if the detrusor muscle of the bladder is behaving itself or contracting in an unstable manner. This takes much of the guesswork out of the situation and is used most often when the doctor cannot decide what is the cause of the incontinence that you are experiencing– unstable bladder, sphincter weakness, nerve damage etc. Generally speaking, video-urodynamics are available in large city hospitals only.

Diathermy: The surgeon can use diathermy through a cystoscope under anaesthesia to remove any polyps that are present or to cauterise any areas on the lining of the bladder that appears to be inflamed.

Surgery: Surgery through the vagina aims at pushing things back into place. Surgery through the abdomen aims at pulling them up and holding them there. The best, long-term surgical results for stress incontinence are achieved via an abdominal approach.

Drugs: These have limited use in the treatment of incontinence but generally aim to do one of the following:

• To quieten down the bladder and stop if from contracting when it shouldn't.
• To increase the bladder capacity.
• To increase resistance in the urethra making it harder for the urine to escape.
• To treat infection or inflammation.
• To provide antihistamines in the presence of allergic reactions within the bladder (when mast cells are present).
• Hormone replacement therapy.

CHAPTER 7

TAKING THINGS INTO YOUR OWN HANDS

S o far this book has looked at the things which can cause problems with your waterworks. Now it is time to get rid of those bad habits which helped you lose control and take on some new ones to put you back in charge. In regaining control of your waterworks, you regain control of your life and knowing that you did it yourself is a great boost to your morale.

When Ya Gotta Go, You Don't Gotta Go

The main symptom of bladder instability is the urgent, knee-crossing, eye watering desire to go. Another is frequency: urinating more than five times a day or more than once at night (nocturia). These symptoms can signify conditions other than pelvic floor weakness such as diabetes or infection so check with your doctor. More commonly, however, these signs can simply be what is called 'a learned response', that is, you taught yourself frequency because of little leaks when you coughed or laughed. The urgency developed later. This response can be unlearned and this simple process is called a Bladder Training Program.

Bladder Training Program

To start the program, you need to make a time/volume chart. Each time you pass water, note the hour and the volume passed. Any measuring jug will do for this purpose. Sometimes, at work for example, it may be inconvenient to measure the volume, so record only the time. However, do try to record both. If you wet yourself, record the letter "W" underneath the time. Daytime means when you are up. Night is any time you are in bed. An example chart is provided on the next page to guide you.

		DAYTIME									NIGHT
MON.	Time	7.30	8.15	10.15	11.30	1.15pm	3.30	5.15	6.30	8.30	12.30
	Vol	350ml 50		150	100	150	100	200	150	175	250
TUES.	Time	7.30 8.45									
	Vol	375 W									
WED.	Time										
	Vol										
THU.	Time										
	Vol										

This chart will show your:
• Minimum volume of urine (50mls in the example).
• Maximum daytime volume of urine (200mls in the example).
• Minimum holding time: day, (45 minutes).
• Maximum holding time: day, (2 hours).
• Overnight volume (250mls).
• Frequency (9 times during the day).

Using the chart to plot your progress, you should now aim for the following approximate goals:
• Minimum volume of 300mls.
• Maximum daytime volume of 500mls.
• Minimum holding time of 3 hours.
• Maximum holding time of 4 hours.
• Frequency of 5 to 8 times per day and once at night.

To achieve these goals, there are several rules to follow:
• Never use the toilet 'just in case'.
• Try not to wear pads.
• Never decrease fluid intake – you should drink at least two litres of water each day.
• Each time you get the urge to go to the toilet, defer for five minutes initially, gradually increasing deferment time as you progress.

Deferring The Urge

Putting off the urge to urinate is the basis of the Bladder Training Program. Each time you want to go to the toilet, follow these steps:

1. Contract the muscles of your pelvic floor (see next chapter for Pelvic Floor Strengthening Program).

2. Apply perineal pressure. Roll up a bath towel and keep it on a chair in the kitchen. Sit on this roll (with the roll running front to back) when you get a

strong urge to urinate. You will need to use perineal pressure until your pelvic floor muscles are strong enough to take over. Then the muscles can be lifted up to fire off the reflex that quietens the unstable bladder contraction. Until the muscles are strong enough you will need to push them up. You can do this by pressing with your hand, using the corner of a table, or using a rolled towel.

3. Use mind games to distract your attention away from your bladder. Some suggestions you might find appropriate include counting backwards from 207 by eights, reciting poetry, doing a crossword. The breathing techniques used in yoga and childbirth preparation classes are also beneficial in keeping your mind off your urgency.

4. Auto-hypnosis or relaxation techniques are useful if you are having trouble getting off to sleep. Try using a relaxation cassette tape. When you can defer every urge to urinate for at least five minutes, progress to holding on for 10 minutes. When you have achieved this goal, increase deferment time to 15 minutes. Do not empty your bladder at the end of the pre-set time unless you still have the urge to go. Gradually, the time between urges increases and your trips to the toilet becomes less frequent. The bladder now only sends "I'm full", messages to the brain when it holds larger urine volumes. This is how urgency fades away gradually: mind over matter.

Setbacks

Take two steps forward and one step back: accept this fact now and the minor setbacks, which are bound to happen, won't have any permanent effect on your program. Memorise the following list of danger periods and when setbacks occur, accept them exactly for what they are: minor hiccups along the way to bladder control. Press on and know you will succeed.
- Rainy, windy days.
- Days when you are tired.
- Those times when you are 'hassled' and not very relaxed.
- When you are run down and, for example, catch a cold.
- Around period time.

Summary

Bladder Training Program.
- Keep a written record of your progress.
- Increase fluid intake to 2 litres per day, avoid drinking alcohol, coffee and too much tea.
- Never go to the toilet just in case.

Defer the urge by:
- Contracting the pelvic floor muscles. Squeeze, lift and hold as long as possible.
- Using perineal pressure.
- Distracting your mind.

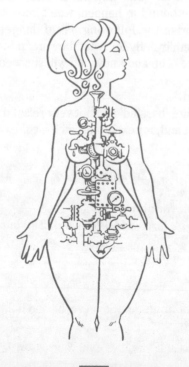

CHAPTER 8

GETTING TO THE CRUX OF THE MATTER

Pelvic Floor Muscle Exercise Program

The ability to control your waterworks depends largely on the ability to control your pelvic floor muscles. If you strengthen these muscles, you should soon regain control of your bladder. In a nutshell, a pelvic floor muscle exercise program follows the 4 Fs:

Feel it working.
Find its limit.
Feel the fast flicks.
Force the limits higher.

Feel It Working

Before you can take action to build up the strength of your pelvic floor muscles, you first have to know if they are working and, if so, how strong they are. To find out if they are working, sit on the toilet with knees wide apart. Start the flow of urine, then stop it. It should stop dead, not just slow to a trickle.

Do not use the urine "stop and start" mechanism as an exercise. Many specialists who work with women who leak urine believe that 'stopping the flow' might cause problems such as urinary retention. If your muscles are weak enough to allow urine leakage under stress (coughing or lifting), then usually are not going to be strong enough for you to feel them contracting unless you are actually using your fingers. Do this first in a supported half-sitting, half-lying position as shown in the diagram. It can be done on the toilet or even standing in the shower, but propping yourself up on a bed is the best position for your first assessment. This position helps to get rid of some of the downward forces that might be pushing on the bladder and pelvic floor.

Place your hand (right or left to suit yourself) as shown in the diagram. Moisten the inserting fingers with saliva or lubricating jelly – do not use

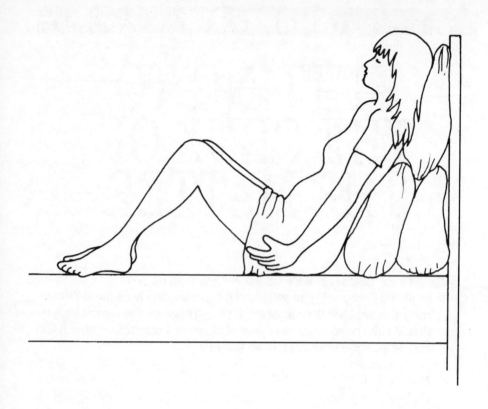

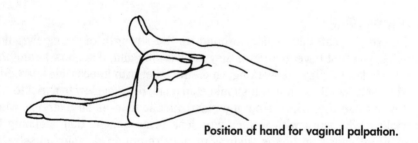

Position of hand for vaginal palpation.

vaseline or face creams as these can irritate the sensitive lining of the vagina – then gently slide your fingers into your vagina. Close your eyes and concentrate. Pull up your muscles as though you need to pass water and can't find a toilet anywhere. Can you feel any movement?

If not, try this: pull up as though you are about to pass wind and the Queen has just walked into the room. Squeeze up to stop the wind from escaping and making a loud embarrassing noise. Don't worry that you are squeezing your back passage rather than your front ... it's impossible to work one without the other at this stage. Still not sure if it's working or not? Then try another trick. Imagine a pin is being brought closer and closer toward your anus (the opening to your back passage). Try to pull this opening away from the pin as it gets closer and closer. Still can't feel anything? Maybe your muscles have been overstretched by childbirth, so now gently push your fingers toward your back passage and try again. While the muscle fibres are being stretched, imagine trying to stop yourself from passing wind. Imagine that pin about to prick your bottom. Don't take your fingers out yet.

While you are in a position to explore these problem points, feel just what happens when you cough – feel the pressure down and the bulging outward. Gently bear down as though opening your bowels and feel the downward movement: this is exactly the opposite feeling to doing a pelvic floor contraction. Now immediately squeeze and pull up – the feeling should be upward and inward with pressure around the back of your fingers. You might feel your cervix, that thing which feels like the tip of your nose, moving up and away from the tips of your fingers. If you still cannot feel a contraction, try placing the index finger of your other hand onto the tip of your tailbone at the back. With the thumb of the hand within your vagina pressing on your public bone at the front, close your eyes again and imagine trying to pull these two points together. Do not hold your breath as this allows you to push down with your diaphragm. Continue to breathe rhythmically in and out as you try to contract your pelvic floor muscles. When you can feel your muscles contracting, no matter how small that contraction is, you are ready to begin your own individually tailored exercise program.

Find Its Limits

In any muscle strengthening program, the aim is to gradually increase the load of work that the muscles are expected to do. The initial load depends on the initial strength of your individual pelvic floor muscles. Working out the basic score of your own pelvic floor muscle puts you in the best position to design an exercise program specially and individually tailored to meet the needs of your own muscles.

Is it working at all? Feel your pelvic floor muscle contract in a squeeze/lift movement. The movement is inwards, a squeeze sensation together with a lifting inward, called a squeeze/lift from here on.

How long you can hold? Next, you need to know exactly how long you can hold the squeeze/lift, measured in 'seconds of hold'. This is easy to measure by counting seconds in a number of ways. You might count by using hundreds, for example, one, one hundred, two, one hundred, three one hundred and so on. Some people count seconds using the words hippopotamus or Mississippi between each number. The point is, how many seconds can you hold a contraction. One second? Three seconds? Five seconds? You will need to remember this number to write it down later. This tells you about the endurance of your pelvic floor muscle.

How many can you do? Next you need to know exactly how many times can you repeat this squeeze and hold. Once? Three times? Six times? This becomes another number for you to remember and write down when you have finished your assessment.

How long in between? How long should you wait between squeeze/lifts? Resting time is extremely important as muscles tire easily. Weak muscles must be given special consideration and time to recover after each contraction. Don't be put off if you can only contract once or twice. This is very often the case and you will be surprised at just how quickly this number will increase. Within your exercise program this initial number of contractions becomes "your number".

How many fast flicks to finish with?

Feel the Fast Flicks

You might recall that pelvic floor muscles are made up of two sets of muscle fibres: fast twitch and slow twitch. So far, the pelvic floor exercises have only addressed the slow twitch component of the pelvic floor muscles. In order to exercise the fast twitch component you need to do a series of fast, hard contractions with no rest in between.

With your fingers in your vagina feel how many quick flicks you can feel before the muscle stops working. Remember, the flicks are meant to be as hard as you can squeeze and as fast as you can squeeze. You will need to keep a record of this number. After you have done each set of your number of squeeze/lift and holds you should finish with a set of fast flick contractions. This makes sure that both the slow twitch fibres of your pelvic floor muscles as well as the fast twitch fibres are being exercised.

Now that your initial assessment is complete, you are ready to begin your own strengthening program. You now know how long in seconds each squeeze/lift should be held for, how many times you should repeat this squeeze/lift/hold and how many quick flicks you should do at the end of each set.

If you have been completely unable to feel anything that vaguely resembles a pelvic floor muscle contraction you will probably need to seek the help of a physiotherapist with special interest and training in this type of therapy.

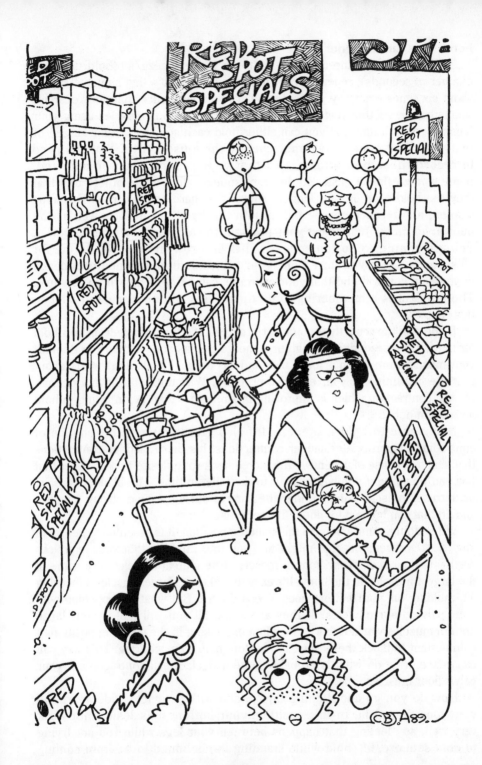

Force This Limit Higher

Taking your baseline numbers try to do your squeeze/lift/hold (for your number of seconds), repeated your number of times. It's that simple! Try this about six times each day. After a few days you will notice that your exercise seems easier. At this stage you will need to retest your muscles using your fingers. You will find that you can either hold each squeeze/lift for longer, or that you can do one or two more before the muscle tires. You will need to record these new numbers so that your program can be adjusted. Some women find it easier to do more squeeze/lifts while others find that they can hold each one for longer. There is no hard and fast rule. For some women, a difference can be felt in both the length of hold as well as the number of times. Just adjust your program to suit your new muscle power. You are aiming to do ten squeeze/lifts in a row, holding each one for 10 seconds. Once you have done your assessment and gained confidence in yourself, you will find that your exercises can be done anywhere, anytime. The problem is remembering to do them. This will be discussed later in this chapter.

If you don't assess, then you can't progress, it's that simple. Can you hold for the full two seconds? A cough or a sneeze can last longer then you think. If your muscle contraction is just a flick and has no hold at all, don't worry about it at the beginning of your exercise program. Wait until you have a definite muscle contraction which is improving in strength – then begin trying to hold for a count of two.

Being able to hold a squeeze/lift also gives you a better chance of controlling inappropriate bladder contractions. It's these bladder contractions that lead to a sense of urgency – the incredibly strong desire to pass water that has you worrying if you will make it to the toilet in time. The bladder muscle, or detrusor muscle, comes under the control during a good strong squeeze and lift that can be held for about five seconds.

When doing contractions in the standing position, it is essential to get rid of any "trick" movements that might fool you into thinking that your exercises are being done well. Your bottom muscles (the gluteal muscles) are some of the largest muscles in the body. It's easy to feel these large muscles squeezing and holding on, your bottom goes nice and hard. But what is happening with your pelvic floor muscles? If they are weak, all you will feel is your large bottom muscles working hard. So, when exercising in the standing position, it is important to block these muscles, to stop them from working. This way you can concentrate on what is probably quite a weak, small contraction of your pelvic floor muscles.

How do you go about doing this? Stand with your feet wide apart and your toes turned in. In this position, your bottom muscles cannot work very well, any feeling that happens between your legs while you are trying to do a squeeze/lift/hold while standing up, is bound to be from coming from your pelvic floor muscle contracting. The trick movements of your buttock and thigh muscles are eliminated if you stand this way. When you have advanced somewhat with your pelvic floor muscle strength, it will not be necessary to stand this way to know that you are exercising effectively in standing.

Easy does it

One thing to remember during your pelvic floor exercise program is that these muscles are under your voluntary control. Just like the muscles in your legs and arms, these muscles can get very tired. Imagine that it is your leg muscles that have not worked properly for years. Your exercise retraining program would be gentle and slow. You wouldn't expect your leg to cope with too much work, you would rest it and not ask it to handle tasks such as a shopping trip in the city followed by a night out with dancing at a nightclub. Think what would happen – your leg would start to ache and swell and it just would not be capable of continuing. Those poor muscles of your pelvic floor deserve just as much tender loving care during their retraining. Please remember to be gentle and don't push them too quickly. You will take two steps forward and one back if you do too much.

Getting "the Knack"

You can see for yourself how much control you can achieve by using a strong squeeze and lift before each cough or sneeze. You might like to try the following simple test. You will need a pencil or ballpoint pen, a couple of pieces of paper towel and a relatively full bladder.

Place the folded hand towel inside your underwear between your legs. While standing with your legs apart, cough hard, three or four times. If you have leaked urine, remove the paper towel and trace in pencil or ballpoint pen around the damp patch on the paper. Now, taking another piece of paper towel, place it as before between your legs and stand with your legs apart. Do a big squeeze/lift and hold at the same time as you cough. Cough as hard as you did before and as many times as you did before. You may notice one of two things. Firstly you may not leak at all. Congratulations – you have the knack! Secondly, if you have leaked, remove the towel and mark the damp patch as before. Chances are the second patch will be much smaller than the first showing that you leaked less urine.

It's important to practice the knack in situations where you usually leak. If you leak during a cough, this has already been explained to you. If you leak when you lift, then you might try a big squeeze/lift and hold before you lift. Likewise, you can try a squeeze/lift and hold while you practice golf swings, serve at tennis or moving from sitting to standing. Practicing the knack is only difficult if you only leak during a sneeze. Sneezing at will is not something most people find easy to do!

Red Spot Specials

Every time you think of it during the day, you should do your number of contractions. Here's a way to help you remember. Buy a packet of small coloured self-adhesive spots (bright red or yellow) and place them strategically throughout the house and at work and even in the car. Every time you notice a spot, do a set of exercises.

Partners Please

It can be quite helpful to ask your partner or some other family member to help you to remember to do your pelvic floor exercises. Explain to them that all that is required is that whenever they think of it, they should ask you "Have you done yours today?".

Here is an example of what your exercise pelvic floor muscle assessment and exercise program might look like.

1. When feeling my pelvic floor squeeze and lift, I feel that the muscle can hold for _____ seconds.
2. I feel that I can repeat this squeeze/lift and hold _____ times.
3. I can feel myself doing _____ quick flicks before the muscle tires.

My personal pelvic floor exercise exercise program.
Whenever I think about it, from three to six times a day I should do:

	Today's Date ___/___/___	Next assessment ___/___/___	Next assessment ___/___/___	Next assessment ___/___/___	Next assessment ___/___/___
Number of squeeze/lifts					
Length of hold in seconds					
Number of quick flicks					

Summary

Muscle Strengthening Plan
- Feel it work.
- Find its limit. Measure and record just what your pelvic floor muscle can do.
- Force this limit higher.
- If you don't assess then you can't progress.
- Do your "red spot specials".
- Get the knack.

Warnings
- Stop your urine flow only once a week only as a test.
- Overdoing your exercises can cause muscle tiredness and temporary loss of control – don't overdo it!
- Expect little progress around your period time – don't give in.
- Whenever you are run down, so is your pelvic floor – don't expect miracles.
- Repeated coughing or sneezing (eg flu or hayfever) can set your program back dramatically – don't be discouraged.
- Remember to try to assess your muscles at the same time each day.

You should notice some change in your urinary habits by the end of one week. It might only be a slight improvement, but this will help keep you on your program. As a general rule, you should aim to manage 10 squeeze/lifts holding each one for 10 seconds from three to six times a day by the end of your program. As you make progress and your number increases, it is time to start using these contractions the way nature intended – as a response to an increase in abdominal pressure. Remember the knack. As part of your program, for some of your number, (for example the first three) you should pull up, cough, relax and encourage your pelvic floor to begin to work again in a reflex manner.

If you think that your pelvic floor muscles are relatively strong, or when you feel you are back in control of your waterworks, it's time to look at a lifelong plan.

Lifetime Plan For Your Pelvic Floor Muscles
- Pull up and hold for six seconds, then relax. Repeat for the entire time you spend in the shower each day.
- Practice the knack before each and every cough or sneeze.
- Do three strong pelvic floor contractions with a five-second hold at the end of every time you have emptied your bladder. Continue to squeeze/lift and hold relax as you wash and dry your hands.
- Repeat your contractions as you prepare each and every cup of tea or coffee.
- Use your PC to stimulate your partner each time you make love.
- Do your red spot specials while you are stopped at any red lights when in the car or standing in line waiting at the supermarket checkout.

CHAPTER 9

SPECIAL HINTS FOR SPECIAL PEOPLE

The Elderly Women

Age is no barrier to success with pelvic floor retraining: old age and incontinence do not have to go hand-in-hand. Everything mentioned so far in this book is very relevant to the elderly woman, but there are a few points that might need to be made clear.

Vaginal Atrophy: The vagina of an elderly woman can be dry, tight and even shallower than that found in many younger women. This is no barrier to assessment. Be careful of the choice of lubricant used on the examining fingers in this situation. Saliva is best, but special lubricating gels (Lubafax, KY) are available from pharmacies if you don't feel happy about using saliva. A fairly new lubricant that has won favour with many women is made from kiwi fruit. In some countries this is sold under the name of 'Sylk'.

General Muscle Condition: The exercise program will tend to be a bit slower in the elderly woman, but probably not as slow as you think. Re-assessment is still advisable at least once a week.

Reaction Time: Urgency, as a urinary symptom, does seem to get worse with age. This, luckily, is no barrier to success with either pelvic floor muscle or bladder training programs.

The Pregnant Woman

Pregnancy is most commonly the start of pelvic floor muscle weakness and therefore very special attention should be paid to this important group of muscles. As soon as pregnancy is confirmed, start an exercise program and stick with it! Assess with your fingers early in the day. Watch the effect of prenatal classes. Do not listen to anyone who tells you that exercises to strengthen the pelvic floor muscles will make delivery more difficult. This is simply not true.

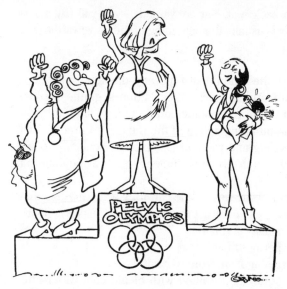

Healthy muscles are strong and resilient, able to cope with the stretching of delivery and then spring back into place almost immediately. Any elite athlete knows that to prepare for a big sporting event, all body muscle groups must be exercised to stretch and strengthen them, otherwise the body is not fit to cope with the gruelling strain of competition. The birth of your baby is probably as close to Olympic competition as you'll ever get, so prepare your body by exercising not only you tummy muscles, but also the muscles of the pelvic floor. Make sure you have a look at your perineum during your pregnancy so you will be able to see the effects that the baby's delivery has had on this part of your body. You will be able to compare your genital area before and after. Don't give up your exercise program if you notice only a small improvement. Remember, during pregnancy all the odds are against you; hormones, the weight of the baby pressing on you bladder and pelvic floor, fatigue levels. If you keep the muscles of the pelvic floor from deteriorating during pregnancy, you will actually be achieving a big improvement. It's just that you won't know about it until after your baby has arrived.

The New Mother

Birth to One Week Later: In the early stages following delivery, your perineal area is likely to feel very tender indeed. Remember that it's not just the skin that has been stretched and maybe torn, the pelvic floor muscles beneath the skin have been stretched too, maybe even badly bruised. If you have had an episiotomy (where the obstetrician or midwife cuts your perineum during delivery of the baby's head), or if you have had a perineal tear, this area is going to feel very fragile indeed. It's not so much painful, but a sensation of tenderness, swelling and weakness. You can feel the lack of tone – everything feels like it might 'fall out'. But take heart – a few simple steps will have your perineum and more importantly, your pelvic floor, back on the road to recovery.

This is a most critical stage in the downfall of the pelvic floor. It's also one of the most emotionally charged stages of your life. While getting to know your new baby and learning to handle it with confidence, it's not hard to let your pelvic floor muscles take a back seat. But be warned ... you will pay a very high price for ignoring them, this is usually the beginning of the downward trend.

Points To Remember

• Rest for 24 hours. This is the amount of time any damaged muscle is allowed to rest – think of the elite athlete again. After 24 hours, gentle exercise of the pelvic floor muscles – in the form of static contractions – should begin, even if stitches are present. The pumping action of the muscle contraction will help get rid of bruising and swelling and will increase blood circulation to and from the damaged tissues with much greater efficiency so that healing can take place as it should.

• Use a mirror to look at your perineum. While carefully watching the area, can you see any movement if you try to contract the muscles of the pelvic floor?

Do not use any form of heat on your perineum.

The best treatment for your perineum is:

1. Soap and water hygiene, rinsing from front to back.

2. You might like to use a squirt bottle filled with clean, cool water after each time you urinate, while you are still sitting on the toilet.

3. Pat dry or use a hairdryer set only on COOL.

4. Ask the nurse to give you an ice pack. Use it for 20 minutes only and repeat every four hours. Ice is more effective the earlier it is used after the baby's birth. It's important to reduce any swelling that might exist around your perineum.

Flow stopping. Again remember, once a week only.

• Keep up your fluid intake. Immediately after the baby is born, you might notice some increase in the amount of urine you pass. This will soon decrease as the water taken into your body is used to produce your milk. This can have the effect of constipating you even more than you already are.

Support your perineum during a bowel motion. Just the thought of using your bowels at this time will be enough to reduce you to a quivering mass of fear and apprehension but, again, take heart. Use a sanitary pad or toilet paper and then gently support the front part of your perineum with your hand. Take a book to the toilet with you, practice your deep breathing and relaxation as well as you can and be assured that this experience need not be all that bad. The simple trick of perineal support will help you over this hurdle.

• On the hour every hour try this simple exercise; pull up the pelvic floor muscle, then cough! Cough gently at first and, as the strength returns to your pelvic floor, push more with your cough. This exercise is designed to make sure you regain the action reflex of your pelvic floor muscles. If you feel that your pelvic floor muscles are very weak in the first weeks after the baby's delivery, you might try crossing your legs and squeezing them together each time you cough or sneeze. This might help to prevent the pelvic floor from being pushed down and causing further damage to nerves and muscles already affected by the delivery.

What was your number of contractions the day before baby was born? Now check what your number is today: you won't be able to use your fingers yet, but you should be able to see the pelvic floor working, or feel it. If not, take three as your number and exercise on the hour, every hour, until you get home to your red spots. It might help to remember the three "T's" – a simple trick for remembering to do your exercises when your red spots are missing. Do your exercises each time you:

Top up the baby.

Turn on a **T**ap.

Go to the **T**oilet.

• Take the load off your pelvic floor. Resting with your feet up won't help the pelvic floor to recover – to take the load off your pelvic floor, you need to lie down. Whenever you are lying down, do some pelvic floor contractions. In this position you won't have to work against all the weight of your abdominal organs and gravity which push downwards on your very weak pelvic floor muscles.

• If you feel tired, so does your pelvic floor. It's possible that the nursing staff in charge of your post-natal recovery will not know much about care for the pelvic floor muscles, although this is changing. The advice given here is that of a professional specifically trained in the field of muscle rehabilitation. Check with a physiotherapist if you have doubts about your post-natal pelvic floor program.

From One Week to One Month After Baby's Birth

It's easy for the new mother to push her own welfare way into the background, but it's vital to your continued well-being that you don't. You have a duty to yourself to regain your pre-pregnant levels of fitness in all areas. There seems no point in exercising your tummy to look good in swimmers if you leak urine every time you cough or sneeze. Settle into the routine of doing your pelvic floor contractions as part of your daily routine. Use the red spot routine to do your number often throughout the day. Again, use the three Ts: toilet, tap and topping up baby, to help you to remember. Check your number each week, at the same time of day. There is likely to be a big difference if you check your number in the morning one week, then try to compare it with a check done late in the evening one week later. Remember to stop flow once a week only.

Breastfeeding mothers may not seem to be getting very far with their exercise program – improvement may be slow or non-existent because low oestrogen levels mean that the pelvic floor muscles are not functioning properly. However, persevere with the program and when your hormone levels return to normal, your pelvic floor muscle tone should improve. When you finish breastfeeding, your pelvic floor will be able to cope as your bladder volumes return to normal. This is especially important if you intend having another baby soon after the first.

CHAPTER 10

PREVENTION IS BETTER THAN CURE

I f we look at all the things mentioned so far that can throw a spanner in your waterworks, then prevention strategy should automatically fall into line. Examine the following list of conditions that are known to be associated with urinary incontinence. It should be clear just which factors might apply to you.

Pregnancy
Vaginal delivery
Being overweight
Pelvic organ prolapse
Constipation
Other bowel symptoms
Chronic cough
Hormones
Drugs
Recurrent urinary tract infections
Childhood bedwetting
Ageing

Your diet can play an important role in the prevention of urinary incontinence. You should aim to follow a nutritional program that will ensure:
• Weight loss if necessary.
• High fibre content to prevent constipation.
• Adequate calcium levels aimed at preventing osteoporosis.

Chronic cough
Stop smoking if this is the cause of your cough. Every time you cough, the pressure is transmitted to your pelvic floor. Chronic chest complaints (eg asthma, bronchitis) will increase your chances of having stress incontinence,

but certainly shouldn't stop you from trying to strengthen your pelvic floor muscles to prevent urine loss.

Drugs
• Speak to your doctor about the effect that your prescribed drugs might be having on your waterworks. Get him/her to review your blood pressure tablets, fluid tablets, sleeping tablets.
• Limit your alcohol intake.
• Limit your caffeine intake through coffee, tea and cola type drinks.

Hormones
See your doctor about the role (if any) that hormone replacement therapy might play in helping your problem. If your ovaries are surgically removed, ensure adequate hormone replacement therapy is continued for a sufficient period of time.

Hints to prevent cystitis
• Keep up your fluid intake – at least two litres each day.
• Always wipe front to back to prevent transferring germs.
• Be careful during lovemaking not to transfer germs from the anus to the vagina.
• Empty your bladder immediately following intercourse.
• Keep your sugar intake low – people with high blood sugar levels tend to suffer recurrent urinary tract infections.
• Avoid bath additives such as bath foam, foaming gel and perfumes.
• Completely empty your bladder every time you go to the toilet.
• Don't hang on for more than six hours.
• Do not use feminine hygiene sprays.
• Use only mild, unperfumed soap on the genital area.
• Avoid using talcum powder between your legs. Talc is an extremely fine powder which can easily irritate the urethra.
• Identify and avoid those foods, if any, which may cause flare-ups.
• Avoid the use of tampons as they can aggravate the urethra. Use sanitary napkins instead.
• Drink a small glass of cranberry juice each day.
• Drink at least two litres of water per day.

The effects of pregnancy, childbirth, menopause and ageing have been discussed. Each of these life stages can play a big part in the downfall of the pelvic floor and its control of your waterworks.

Stop The Problem Before It Starts
In taking charge of your pelvic floor muscles and your bladder habits, you take charge of your waterworks. Use this book to lead yourself to a drier future full of self-esteem, happy in the knowledge that you were able to help yourself.

Where Can I Go For Help?

Your Local Doctor: Can arrange tests to ensure that you are not suffering from symptoms that require help other than a bladder training program or a pelvic floor strengthening program. If necessary, your doctor can arrange to refer you to a specialist for a consultation, further investigations and management.

Your Physiotherapist: Contact the Chartered Society of Physiotherapy, telephone 020 7242 1941.

The Continence Foundation:
307 Hatton Square
16 Baldwin Gardens
London
EC1N 7RJ
Helpline: 0845 345 0165

CHAPTER 11

PELVIC FLOOR EXERCISES: THE BELLS AND WHISTLES

W hen people are serious about exercising, they often use equipment to help them as they work. The equipment might take the form of complicated weight and pulley systems like those used in gymnasiums on exercise 'circuits'. The equipment might take the form of special walking or rowing machines or a bicycle, or something as simple as a set of weights that are carried as you walk. The equipment is designed to do a number of things to help your general exercise programe. Firstly, it helps to increase the effectiveness of your program. Secondly, it can in some cases let you see just how you are improving, how close you are getting to your goal. Thirdly, equipment also often helps to keep you motivated and focused on your goals.

A good pelvic floor exercise program is really no different and there are quite a few pieces of equipment available to help as you go. Some of the equipment is available for purchase and personal use, while other equipment is generally used by the healthcare professionals involved in the management of poor pelvic floor muscle control and/or urinary incontinence. The rest of this chapter will provide you with explanations of the most commonly used exercise appliances.

It is important to remember that none of these appliances are 'stand alone'. Each and every one of them is designed to play only a part in an exercise program. There is no substitute for a well designed exercise programe. The appliances mentioned here simply help your basic program – they are an addition to it.

BioFEEDBACK

Biofeedback might be defined as using some sort of message (lights buzzers, graphs etc) to tell you about a body system that you are usually unaware of. A good example of this is as simple as your bathroom scales. The scales tell you by numbers, just how much your body weighs. Biofeedback machines are used to give you feedback about just how well your pelvic floor muscles are working. The most convenient and the cheapest form of biofeedback has already been discussed – using your own fingers within your vagina. (See chapter 8 – Getting to the Crux of the Matter.)

The EDUCATOR ®

This simple device can be used firstly to see if your pelvic floor muscles are working correctly, i.e. pulling upwards and not pushing down, and secondly, to show you how much movement of the pelvic floor muscles is taking place each time you do a squeeze and lift. If the EDUCATOR® does not move at all, it is a good sign that your pelvic floor muscles need some working on!

The EDUCATOR® consists of a small plastic vaginal probe which has a very thin indicator or 'wand' attached to it. When the probe part is placed within the vagina, the 'wand' should sit outside and in such a position that it can be easily seen extending upwards between the thighs. During a pelvic floor muscle squeeze, if you are using your muscles correctly, the indicator will move *downwards*. If the indicator part of the probe moves *upwards* (towards you) this means that you are pushing with your tummy muscles and *not* squeezing your pelvic floor muscles against the probe.

The correct movement of your pelvic floor muscles is very important if you are to be able to get 'the knack'. A good 'squeeze and lift' will tilt the indicator part of the EDUCATOR® downwards and away from you and as your muscles improve their performance you should notice the arc of the movement increasing. The EDUCATOR® may also be used to help increase the time you can hold a contraction. Just count the number of seconds the indicator is held down, it will drift back upwards to its original position as soon as your muscles tire. You can use it to exercise by doing slow, 'holding' contractions or quick 'flick' exercises that can help prevent leakage during a cough or sneeze.

Perineometers

These are biofeedback machines which are relatively inexpensive and available for your own personal use. These are small hand-held devices that have a probe, which fits easily into the vagina. As pelvic floor muscles squeeze against the probe, there is an immediate increase in pressure. You can see just how much pressure the muscles are exerting as they work. You can also clearly see exactly how long you can hold your pelvic floor muscle squeeze before the muscle begins to tire. As well as this, how many repetitions your muscle is capable of doing in each set, can easily be seen.

As with all exercise equipment, it is really important that the perineometer is actually measuring pelvic floor squeeze pressure and nothing else. If you place a pressure perineometer within your vagina, hold it in place with your hand, and bear down as if using your bowels, you will get a pressure increase on the vaginal probe which will not be coming from pelvic floor muscle squeeze. When using any portable, hand held perineometer, it is quite easy to make sure that you are squeezing and not pushing. Simply place the probe within your vagina and try to do a pelvic floor muscle squeeze. If you are in fact using your pelvic floor muscles, the outside end of the probe will tilt downward, or you might see an inward movement of the probe as if your muscles are pulling the probe deeper into your vagina. If the outside end of the probe moves upwards, or if it moves as though it is going to come out of your vagina, this means that you are pushing with your tummy muscles and not squeezing your pelvic floor muscle against the probe (see 'the educator' at the beginning of this chapter). If this is the case, it might be better for you to use your fingers for a little while longer to be sure that you pelvic floor muscles are indeed working, and that you are not bearing down. Healthcare professionals specially trained in this area will be able to help you if you just don't seem to be able to get it right.

Healthcare professionals themselves use a couple of different methods of biofeedback in order to get the best performance possible from your pelvic floor muscles. These might include pressure biofeedback as we have already discussed, or they might use EMG biofeedback (electromyographic biofeedback). 'Electro' meaning that the vaginal probe doesn't register pressure, it registers tiny electrical impulses sent out by the muscles of the pelvic floor as they contract. 'Myo' meaning muscle, and 'graphic' meaning that the output from the muscle is displayed so that you can clearly see it. These professionally used machines are often connected to a computer and a screen. As you carry out your pelvic floor muscle exercise program, your progress can easily be followed and easily printed out so that very accurate records of your progress can be kept.

Exercising the muscles of your pelvic floor using a perineometer

In the same way that has been described for using your fingers to feel the pelvic floor muscle work – the perineometer can provide you with an accurate readout of exactly how long you should hold each contraction, and how many contractions you should do in each set. Again, care should be taken not to tire the muscles by making sure that there is adequate rest time between each contraction. As a rule of thumb, you should rest for twice as long as you hold. For example, if you can hold each contraction for four seconds, you should rest for about eight seconds before doing your next contraction. Remember – you are aiming to be a perfect – able to hold each muscle squeeze for ten seconds and to do ten squeezes in a set. The perineometer will also give the same information about your 'flick' contractions. How many you should to do in each set will be clearly shown by the perineometer.

With the very accurate information to hand provided by the perineometer about your pelvic floor muscles, you can repeat your individual exercise set any time you remember. The exercises that you do throughout the day are still a very important part of your exercise program. The perineometer tells you just how well you are going. Your regular exercise sets are what will move you forward to the next level.

Weighted Vaginal Cones

Yet another form of biofeedback is provided by the use of vaginal weights. Because these are cone shaped, they are sometimes referred to as vaginal cones. Cones can be sold in sets of about five cones, each cone being slightly heavier than the last, or in a set that provides you with the ability to open the cone and insert the weight of your choice within it. These particular cones (those that can be added to or subtracted from) can also be sterilised in an autoclave. The sets of cones each of different weights are sold for individual use and cannot be re-sterilised.

Cones work in two ways. Firstly as the cone tries to slip out of your vagina, the muscles of the pelvic floor have to squeeze and lift to keep the cone from falling out. This is a very accurate muscle action; it encourages both squeeze and lifts, which is the normal way the pelvic floor muscles should work. Also, cones are used while you are standing up. This is the position in which you are more likely to use your pelvic floor muscles in real life, to prevent 'accidents'. Secondly, cones work because they make the pelvic floor muscles work against the resistance of the weight of the cone. Pumping iron for the pelvic floor muscles. Resistance is important whenever muscle strength needs to be increased and cones provide the resistance very effectively. Cones are often recommended for use when there is no access to trained healthcare professionals. Sometimes, when a woman has a very large vagina, the cones might be inserted and simply sit sideways within the vagina. In cases such as this, the women using the cones would have no sensation of 'oops – its going to slip out!' and it should be obvious to her that something wasn't quite right.

Healthcare professionals are constantly working to develop and provide simple and effective methods of measuring pelvic floor muscle function. A well-trained healthcare professional should always provide you with a clear description of how the measuring instrument works and exactly what it is measuring.

USEFUL ADDRESSES

PHYSIOTHERAPY GROUPS

The Chartered Society
of Physiotherapy
14 Bedford Row
London WC1R 4ED
Tel: 020 7242 1941

Association of
Chartered
Physiotherapists in
Obstetrics and
Gynaecology
c/o The Chartered
Society of
Physiotherapy
14 Bedford Row
London WC1R 4ED
Tel: 020 7242 1941

Chartered
Physiotherapists
Promoting Continence
Jane Dixon
Secretary CPPC
Montagu Clinic
Ouse Valley House
Station Road
St. Ives
PE27 5BH
Tel: 01480 460 049
Fax: 01480 461 145
e-mail:
dixonj@waitrose.com

The Organisation of
Chartered
Physiotherapists in
Private Practice
Cedar House
Bell Plantation
Watling Street
Towcester
Northants
NN12 6HN
Tel: 01327 354 441
Fax: 01327 354 476
e-mail:
towcesterphysio@aol.com

SOURCES OF INFORMATION AND HELP

The Continence Foundation
307 Hatton Square
16 Baldwins Gardens
London EC1N 7RJ
Helpline: 0845 345 0165
Fax: 020 7404 6876
e-mail: continence-help@
dial.pipex.com
www.continence-foundation.
org.uk

Incontact
United House
North Road
London N7 9DP
Tel: 020 7700 7035
e-mail:
info@incontact.org
www.incontact.org
*A charity that provides
information and support
for people affected by
bowel and bladder
problems*

Enuresis Resource
and Information
Centre (ERIC)
34 Old School House
Brittania Road
Kingswood
Bristol BS15 8DB
Tel: 0117 960 3060
*Provides advice on
bedwetting, soiling and
daytime bedwetting for
parents, children and
professionals*

Alzheimers Society
Gordon House
10 Greencoat Place
London
SW1P 1PH
Tel: 020 7306 0606
*Provides information
sheets on incontinence*

Stroke Association
Whitecross Street
London EC1Y 8JJ
Tel: 020 7566 0300

Association for
Continence Advice
102A Astra House
Arklow Road
New Cross
London SE14 6EB
Helpline: 020 8692 4680
e-mail:
info@aca.uk.com
www.aca.uk.com
*membership organization
for healthcare professionals
only.*